One Woman's Path To Health

A Guide to Healthy Living

One Woman's Path To Health

A Guide to Healthy Living

Tricia McAvoy

One Woman's Path to Health: A Guide to Healthy Living
By Tricia McAvoy

Published by:
> Pueblo Press
> 131 Daniel Webster Highway #325
> Nashua, NH 03060

Front Cover Design, Tricia McAvoy
Back Cover Photo, Heidi Waddell
Interior Design by Mark Roberts, Taos Press

Requests for permission should be sent to:
> Pueblo Press
> 131 Daniel Webster Highway #325
> Nashua, NH 03060
> 860-303-8772

ISBN: 978-0-692-63660-2

Dedication

I dedicate this book in gratitude to Stephen Dutka, owner of The Natural Food Store in Niantic, CT, who greatly influenced my thinking about organic food, natural healing and a non-toxic household. And to all my teachers in yoga and life, I thank you.

Contents

Acknowledgments

I deeply thank my dear friends and mentors who have supported me in following my dreams. It is an amazing feeling to be able to accomplish this task and I could not have done it alone.

"It does not matter how slowly you go as long as you do not stop."

~ Confucius ~

PREFACE

I am writing this book with the intention that it is a jumping off point for many into the pool of healthy living. The information included has been a result of my direct experience over the past 20 years of my life. I did not make all these changes at once, nor do I recommend that for you. Simply take in the information provided here and let it inform you.

Making change is never easy and it is always best to take small steps in the direction you wish to go. When I feel overwhelmed, I tend to freeze and do nothing. Take this information as one step in the direction of healthier living. We are all responsible to find our own path in life, be gentle with yourself as you move towards making lasting changes for yourself.

Tricia McAvoy
Trishbliss.com

"When society finally discovers that refined sugar is just another white powder, along with pure cocaine, it will change its mind and attitude toward refined food addiction."

~ Dr. Serge Ahmed ~

CHAPTER 1

The Sweet Stuff Isn't So Sweet

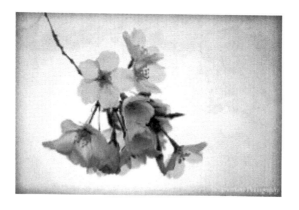

One of my earliest childhood memories is hoisting myself up onto the kitchen counter and going into the cupboard to find the sugar bowl with my mother yelling from the other room, "Tricia, are you in the cupboard again?" "Noooooooo," I yelled back as I scampered down as quietly as possible. I was addicted to sugar at a very young age (as sadly, many others are as well). Nobody thought of it as an addiction back then though. I would literally eat spoonfuls of sugar from the jar to satisfy my cravings if there wasn't another option in the house. I grew up in the 1970's, at a time which some might deem as the beginning of the junk food age in America.

I was a classic American kid, totally influenced by advertisements on the television for toys and breakfast cereals. I ate a diet consisting mostly of processed foods, soda, canned vegetables and cube steak. Oh, and candy, I ate a whole lot of candy. I probably had ten cavities in my baby teeth and began getting them pretty quickly when my adult teeth appeared as well.

I didn't know what an impact all that junk food would have on my health (mental and physical) and frankly I could not have cared less. I just wanted my fix. I loved going down to the neighborhood store where my dad brought me before our weekly visit to the movies. He would give me a dollar and with that I could get two candy bars. I remember how hard it was to only pick two kinds but generally I left with my favorites, a Butterfinger and the classic $100,000 Bar.

I ate more than two candy bars a week

though. I had the stuff everyday, all day, all the way from breakfast to an after-dinner snack before bed. And if I didn't have any sugar, I was mighty upset. I would rage and scream and cry. Looking back, I have more compassion for my little self, hooked on the white stuff, but I also see how hard it must have been to live with me then!

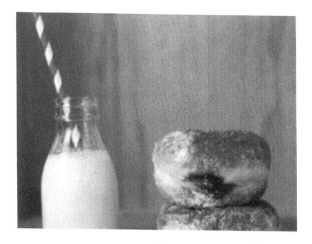

Sugar is an issue. And these days, people are starting to talk about it and write about it and educate themselves on the truth of it. There is even an episode of *The Simpsons* from January 2002 titled, "Sweet and Sour Marge," that recognizes the depth of the problem with a bit of humor. And the depth of the problem is in realizing that sugar is indeed a dangerous drug.

Dr. Serge Ahmed at the University of Bordeaux, France, has found that it may be as addictive as cocaine since 94% of his laboratory rats have been shown to prefer sugar or saccharin over intravenous cocaine![1] If you search on Amazon you will find a variety of books to help you overcome a sugar addiction.

But why would anyone ever want to give up sugar? It tastes so good, I agree! But the long and short of it is that it is wreaking havoc on your health, physically and mentally.

Sugar overdosing had long affected my personality, whether I wanted to admit it or not. I remember one specific day when I was still in college and after being particularly nasty to my boyfriend I thought, "Maybe, I'm just an angry person and that is how I am going to be forever." That was a sad day. At the time, I had no idea that the amount of sugar I was consuming was having a chemical effect on my body and making me quite

---

[1] Connie Bennett, "The Rats Who Preferred Sugar Over Cocaine" *Huffington Post Blog* (November 17, 2011) http://www.huffingtonpost.com/connie-bennett/the-rats-who-preferred-su_b_712254.html

inpatient and irritable with a very short fuse. I'd just explode in a rage for little reason at all.

Later in life, when I had removed all forms of sugar from my diet for a year, I found that I was actually a much nicer person than I had ever imagined! And when I welcomed the sugar back into my life after that year of abstinence, it also became blatantly clear how much my personality could be affected by too much sugar in my system.

Sugar comes in many different forms these days. In my opinion, the most dangerous of them all is *high fructose corn syrup*. Throw away anything in your pantry that has that ingredient included, for it is truly detrimental to your health. High fructose corn syrup is quickly absorbed into the bloodstream and goes directly to the liver, which then kicks in your fat production.

Why Balancing Blood Sugar is Crucial to Good Health

The latest buzzword out in the medical fields is *INFLAMMATION*, and guess what? Yup, sugar is one cause of inflammation in your body. Blood sugar refers to the quantity of glucose in the blood at any given time.

People didn't give much concern to blood
sugar until *Time* magazine came out with a
headline story in 2004 titled, "The Secret
Killer: The Surprising Link between
Inflammation and Heart Attacks, Cancer,
Alzheimer's and Other Diseases." [2]

We eat sugar and we feel good for a while
but then the body crashes and you need more
to pick you up again. When blood sugar goes
high and then low and then high again
throughout the day, it causes cellular
inflammation to occur in the body. Although
this cellular inflammation is below the
perception of pain in the body, it is the number
one cause to many chronic health conditions.[3]
Sugar consumption is now linked to both
inflammation and weight gain. The good
news, however, is that diet can help control
inflammation in the body.

Has sugar had a grip on you for too long? The

---

[2] Christine Gorman, Alice Park and Kristina Dell, "The Secret
Killer: The Surprising Link between Inflammation and Heart
Attacks, Cancer, Alzheimer's and Other Diseases" *Time* (February
23, 2004)
*http://content.time.com/time/magazine/article/0,9171,993419,00.ht
ml*
[3] Barry Sears, MD, "What is Cellular Inflammation?" *Zone Labs
Blog* (January 10, 2012)
http://www.zonediet.com/blog/what-is-cellular-inflammation/

first step may feel like the most difficult, but you don't need to be alone in the journey. When you are ready to take the first step toward releasing the grip of sugar, I'm here for you. Simply reach out to me at trishbliss@me.com.

"Life is precious and you are precious, so treat yourself accordingly."

~ Libby Weaver ~

CHAPTER 2

Feeling Betrayed

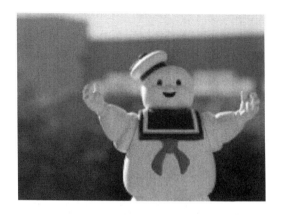

When I was 9 years old, my beloved teacher Mr. Lozelle, made a comment during the 4th grade assembly that if I didn't watch out I would have to start going to Weight Watchers with him. I didn't know what Weight Watchers was at the time, but none the less, I was still humiliated. My sugar addiction had gotten the better of me by then and my small body system couldn't handle the overload of glucose in my body, so it started turning it into fat.

I had some emotional hardships that went along with my compulsive eating behavior, including my sisters and brothers leaving one by one for college and then my parents' divorce that soon followed. Food had become a safe and trusted friend, one that wouldn't leave me or let me down. But my body started turning on me, it had had enough abuse and could no longer tolerate my eating habits.

It is hard being a chubby kid ~ the ridicule, the shame, it stays with you long after you grow. I'm still trying to reprogram my brain to stop calling myself *FAT*. For so many years I had unconsciously repeated to myself, "I'm fat. I'm fat. I'm fat," even when I wasn't overweight in my body, I was still overweight in my mind. Or never thin enough. Holding a distorted body image of oneself can also impact your health. I was constantly striving for a better body with thinner thighs and a more toned stomach, but in reality I simply just hated myself.

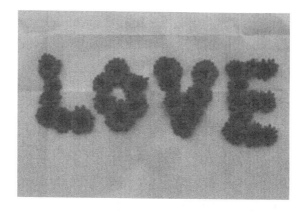

The way you think about yourself and your body has a direct impact on your health. Maybe it does not happen immediately, but it definitely has long-term effects. I started gaining weight as a young person and I hated my body for most of my life. I felt like a victim and that it was all out of my control. I felt sorry for myself because I wasn't born with a different body type, like many of my friends who could eat whatever they wanted and never gain a pound.

When I woke up and finally took personal responsibility for my thoughts and my actions, things began to change for me. The body is a super-healing machine, but many feel that their body has betrayed them. Did you know that cells and tissues in your body regenerate every day? The stomach lining is renewed every 5 days, skin cells once a month, the liver every 6 weeks and your bones every 3 months.[4] So what keeps us the same? It's our thoughts, our belief systems, and the things we repeat to ourselves every single day about how things are for us. Otherwise, we would be creating ourselves anew all the time!

Changing your thoughts starts with self-awareness. What is it that you repeat to yourself every day? With what ideas or beliefs are you identifying? Being able to stop and create time and space for you to concentrate and contemplate and really do some deep listening is a key to gaining self-awareness. This practice didn't start for me until I was many years older, but you can start right away.

---

[4] Howard Murad, MD, "The Water Secret: The Cellular Breakthrough to Look and Feel 10 Years Younger" (2010)

You can begin by setting aside as little as 10 minutes every day. Starting small is the best way to insure success. If you place the bar too high, you'll be setting yourself up for disappointment. This is about creating a new habit. You are worth 10 minutes every day!

Interested in exercises to shift your mindset for lasting results? I've got some great tools to help, send me an e-mail and put "Mindset Exercises" in the subject line. trishbliss@me.com.

"The number one problem most patients (people) face is the inability to love themselves."

~ Bernie Siegal ~

CHAPTER 3

The Day Chronic Disease Arrived

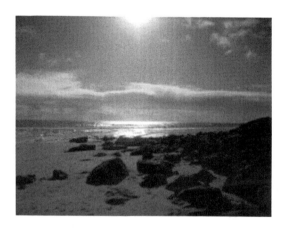

In the summer of my 15th year, I was at the beach on the Rhode Island coastline with my sister. It was a hot and humid day and I was in the ocean playing in the waves when I suddenly felt like I got the wind knocked out of me. I couldn't breathe and as I staggered out of the water, I saw my sister running down the beach with a towel in her hands.

I must have looked awful because she wrapped me up tight and sat me right down on the sand by the water's edge. I remember her rocking me and telling me I was going to be all right.

That was my first autoimmune response. My whole body had swollen up and I was deathly white and covered in red blotches ~ something was definitely wrong. The specialist diagnosed me with Rheumatoid Arthritis and prescribed some anti-inflammatory medications. Two years later I was diagnosed with Systemic Lupus Erythematosus (SLE), which is an autoimmune disease in which the body's immune system mistakenly attacks itself. It can affect the joints, kidneys, brain and other organ systems as well as the skin. When the doctor gave me the Lupus diagnosis, my mother who was a Registered Nurse her whole life, burst into tears in his office. I didn't know what Lupus was, but I knew for certain that it was not good news.

But I was heading to college with my whole life ahead of me. For a few months I played the card, *I have a life-threatening autoimmune disease* to gain sympathy but that quickly got old. My other sister had gifted me a book about one woman's experience with Lupus and let me tell you, it was just terrible. She was sick all the time, couldn't go out in the sun, and was constantly in pain. I think it was the very first book that I closed halfway through and refused to finish. It had become blatantly clear to me that Lupus was not what I signed up for in this life and I made a vow to myself that day that I was going to find a way to heal my body and regain my health.

Lupus and Rheumatoid Arthritis are just two of a very long list of autoimmune diseases that have begun to surface in mass quantities. Ultimately, every autoimmune disorder is a result of inflammation on a cellular level and occurs when the immune system has been overtaxed for an extended length of time.

A healthy body has an immune system that turns on to fight invaders and then turns off again when the danger has been controlled. But autoimmune disease causes a mutation within the cells and the body believes that its own cells are invaders and begins to attack them.

In some people the body attacks the joints, in others the liver, and still in others the nervous system. It has yet to be determined why each body chooses its unique form of attack, but ultimately all these diseases root back to one common cause, poor health in the gut which is directly linked to the quality of food you choose to eat. To understand this a bit more, let me share a little of what I've learned about gut health.

"Own your story, write the ending."

~ Brene Brown

CHAPTER 4

What's The Big Deal About Gut Health?

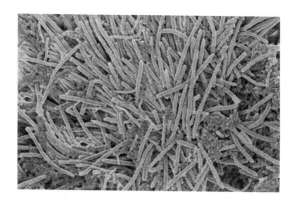

The gut is actually your whole digestive system from the top of the esophagus to the anus and is also known as the gastrointestinal tract or the alimentary canal. It contains 60% of the cells in your body (that is significant) and has more neurons than the spine itself, with 100 million neurons embedded in its walls.[5] It has also been

---

[5] Liz Lipski, PhD, CCN, CNS, LDN,

recently discovered that 95% of serotonin in the body is found the gastrointestinal tract.[6] Serotonin is a mood regulator that has been found to impact every type of behavior we have as human beings including our appetites, digestion, sleep, memory and sexual desire and function.

We also now know that stress can impact the body through the intestinal tract. When you live in a constant state of stress (internal and external), your gut health is greatly affected.

The gut also contains what scientists are now calling "the second brain" or the enteric nervous system. This second brain processes emotions and sends a direct signal to the brain in our head.[7] If you have felt "butterflies in your stomach," that is one indication of this highly sensitive system which has been linked to recent discoveries of the vagus nerve's functions. 90% of the fibers in the vagus nerve

---

[6] Adam Hadhazy, "Think Twice: How the Gut's 'Second Brain' Influences Mood and Well- Being," *Scientific* American (February 12, 2010) *http://www.scientificamerican.com/article/gut-second-brain/*

[7] Adam Hadhazy, "Think Twice: How the Gut's 'Second Brain' Influences Mood and Well- Being," *Scientific* American (February 12, 2010) *http://www.scientificamerican.com/article/gut-second-brain/*

carry information from the gut to the brain and back down again, so it is indeed a super highway connecting the two brains.[8]

It is also important to note that 70% of your immune system is also located in your gut. So in actuality, the health of your gut impacts the health of your whole being ~ physical, mental and emotional. This is big news!

The other latest news relating to our gut is that essentially, we are only 10% human![9] Believe me, I know how crazy that sounds. Have you heard the term microbiome yet? 90% of the cells in our body are actually non-human cells, they are bacterial cells located mostly in the gut lining of the colon but also on the surface of the skin. Yes, this is a good thing as we would not be alive without our bacterial friends helping us along!

Your intestines carry approximately 4000 different species of bacteria and fungi, numbering upwards of 100 trillion! And we actually need all of these little bugs in order to stay alive. But know that there is a difference between good bacteria and bad bacteria. If you have an overgrowth of yeast or bad bacteria, it

---

[8] Vagus Nerve: *https://en.wikipedia.org/wiki/Vagus_nerve*

[9] Alanna Collin, "10% Human" (Harper Collins, 2015)

can create a myriad of problems with your digestion as well as your emotions. It can even lead to cravings for foods that aren't good for you. Those little microorganisms can send messages to your brain (via the vagus nerve) saying, "I want more sugar! I want more flour! I want more dairy products and simple carbohydrates that can easily turn into sugar! Feed me!"

But when is inflammation a good thing? Your body creates inflammation around areas that need healing. When you get cut or sprain an ankle, the body creates space around the wound so that it can heal effectively. Your body is such an amazing machine to contemplate! It is when the immune system is constantly bombarded with so-called alien particles that it goes into overdrive, which causes cellular inflammation.

This cellular inflammation is the still yet undetectable red flag of poor health. Unfortunately, there is no way yet to determine cellular inflammation in the body, we only know about it when it progresses to another stage of inflammation that can attack any one (or more) of the body's systems to cause a more serious disease.

"Believe you can and you're halfway there."

~ Theodore Roosevelt ~

CHAPTER 5

Finding a New Way

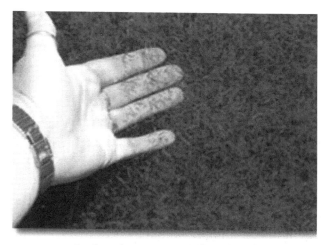

Aphanizomenon Flos-Aquae

At age 25 I was extremely unhappy, I was 50 pounds overweight and I was clueless on what I wanted to do as a career. Purely by grace, that same year I was introduced to both yoga and blue green algae. Aphanizomenon flos-aquae (AFA) or as it is commonly known, Blue Green Algae, is considered by many to be the very first living, breathing organism on planet Earth, with fossil remains dating back to 3.4 BILLION years ago.[10] They are said to be the first organisms to release oxygen into the atmosphere back then and through the process of evolution, some believe all life forms may have originated from these tiny thread-like beings.

As it was introduced to me, I found that blue green algae contains a variety of phytonutrients such as chlorophyll and carotenoids as well as polyunsaturated fatty acids that promote good health in the body. Another amazing fact about blue green algae is that it has an almost identical amino acid profile as that of the human body, along with a full spectrum of vitamins (except D & E) and minerals in trace amounts, which makes it 100% assimilated by the body.[11] And, on top of that, it is also made of 60% protein, a true super food! From the stories I heard of other peoples' success with the algae, I decided to give it a try. I had been taking the anti-inflammatory medications for 10 years at that point, with little success. I still had swollen

---

[10] "Ancient Alga Fossil Most Complex Yet", *Science News*, Vol. 108, 20 September 1975, p. 181)

[11] Robert Alan Ross, "Nature's First Raw Super Food" *http://www.rawfoodlife.com/natures_first_raw_superfood.html*

fingers almost daily, and I still got physically ill if I had too much sun exposure. I was ready to find a new way to heal myself.

As mentioned in Chapter 3, thoughts and beliefs are an important part of the healing process. I totally believed that the blue green algae would help me. Since I was certain that it was my answer to regaining my health and my life, I wouldn't let anyone else tell me differently. I spent a whole lot of money on the algae that first year and at one time I was taking 20 capsules daily but I deeply believed it was helping me.

After just one full year on the algae, my blood work showed that the anti-DNA antibody (which is one indication of Lupus) came up negative! My rheumatologist told me that it was very unusual for that to happen and that was all that I needed to hear, I slowly weaned myself off of my medications and haven't looked back since.

I believe the Blue Green Algae helped to rebuild my immune system, but that is not the end of my story.

Percentage of Water in Your Parts

Bones 22%

Muscles 70%

Brain 73%

Blood 80%

Lungs 90%

"Own your story, write the ending."

~ Brene Brown ~

CHAPTER 6

The Elixir of Life

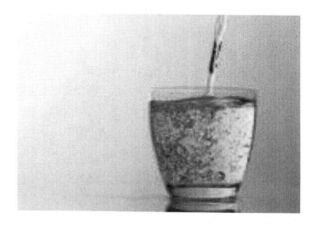

A round the time that I started taking the algae products, I also started drinking copious amounts of water. It was explained to me that drinking the water would help toxins flush out of my body, so I got up to about a gallon a day (which is probably too much for anyone). It actually diluted my urine so much that I had to retake a drug test for an insurance company I was applying to three times before I passed.

There is such a thing as too much of a good thing. If you drink too much water, too fast it can also dilute sodium levels in the bloodstream and cause water intoxication and an imbalance of water in the brain.

But in moderation, water is an essential component of life and good health. Over 60% of your body is made of water (80% in infants) and water truly encourages the health of each and every cell in the body. Water is so necessary for so many body functions including digestion, immune function, blood flow, the synthesizing of protein and also regulating your core body temperature. It increases metabolism and regulates appetite to help maintain a healthy body weight as well.

Water naturally hydrates the skin and gives it a healthy glow by ensuring proper cellular formation. It also prevents constipation and is essential for circulation in the body.[12]

We've all heard the recommendations to drink 8 glasses of water daily. You can live a month without food but only one week without water. And while drinking water is always important, it is good to get some of

---

[12] Howard Murad, MD, "The Water Secret: The Cellular Breakthrough to Look and Feel 10 Years Younger" (2010)

your water through your food as well ~ meaning your fruits and vegetables. Because it takes a while for the cell walls of the produce to break down during digestion, the water is able to be absorbed more slowly than when you quickly drink a glass of water.[13]

Water carries with it essential vitamins and minerals wherever it travels. So caffeinated beverages do not count as water intake because caffeine actually dehydrates your body by preventing water from traveling to where it is needed in the body. By the time you feel thirsty, your body has already lost a percentage of water, so be sure to stay hydrated so that you don't stress yourself out (literally) with mild dehydration. Often fatigue during the day can be this mild state of dehydration.

So now what's the scoop on chlorinated water? These days federal regulations require that water supplied to suburban and urban areas of the U.S. is run through a treatment plant where it is pumped full of chlorine. Granted, the chlorine has helped stave off many infectious water borne illnesses and so has in fact saved many lives, but still it is not

---

[13] Howard Murad, MD, "The Water Secret: The Cellular Breakthrough to Look and Feel 10 Years Younger" (2010)

the healthiest thing we can do for ourselves. In
Europe, several countries have implemented
ways to oxidize water without the use of
chlorine.[14]

Chlorine has drying effects on the hair and
skin but more importantly it is absorbed
through the skin and into the body when
showering, bathing or swimming in
chlorinated water. When showering, skin
pores widen more readily and allow more
chlorine to enter your body. It is said that one
will absorb and inhale more chloroform (the
vaporous form of chlorine) in a 10-minute
shower than by drinking 8 glasses of the same
water.[15]

But that doesn't mean drinking it is a good
idea either. By oxidizing lipid contaminants in
the water, chlorine creates free radicals in our
bodies.[16] Free radicals are highly reactive ions
that lack a positive electron and while these

[14] "Alternatives to Chemical Disinfection of Drinking Water,"
February 1999, http://www.fwr.org/waterq/dwi0808.htm
[15] Danica Collins, "Dangers of Chlorine in Your Shower,"
Underground Health Reporter,
http://undergroundhealthreporter.com/dangers-of-chlorine-in-
your-shower/#axzz3yvwFjsqk
[16] Joseph G. Hattersley, "The Negative Health Effects of
Chlorine," The Journal of Orthomolecular Medicine (Vol. 15, 2nd
Quarter 2000)

are a necessary part of our body, when they are in excess they can lead to disease and chronic disease. Chlorine also creates oxysterols, which are formed when oxygen and lipid molecules combine. Cholesterol is an oxysterol and it serves a positive function in the body, again, just not in excess. Too many oxysterols and free radicals can harm the arteries and may initiate cancer growth.

Chlorine also destroys beneficial bacteria in the gut such as Acidophilis, which is a friendly bacteria living in the lining of the colon and a fundamental part of a strong immune system.[17]

---

[17] Kristen Michaelis, "Chlorinated Showers & Baths Kill Gut Flora," Food Renegade, *http://www.foodrenegade.com/chlorinated-showers-baths-kill-gut-flora/*

"There is no social change without personal change."

~ Deepak Chopra ~

CHAPTER 7

Reality Check

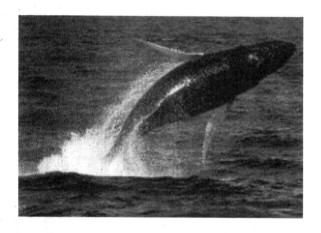

During no part of this process has it been easy for me. Today, some people hold a picture of me as a healthy and vibrant being and believe that I have been that way all my life. They also assume my success at recovering my own health has been a "piece of cake" (ha ha) for me. However, that is not the case. I have fought every step towards better health, and yet I have kept on my path because I definitely want to live in a healthy body that is free of aches and digestive issues every day.

Change is not easy for anyone and changing habits is one of the hardest things to accomplish. But remember, small moves are the best way to make lasting change in life.

Another important factor in my desire to make significant change in my eating was watching my father slowly die from complications of diabetes. My dad was not grossly overweight, but he had a big belly. Doctor after doctor had recommended for him to make change in his diet, but his genoa salami grinders and pepperoni pizza were more important to him than his life. By the end of his days, he had to have several sections of his legs removed and could no longer walk on his own. That was another big wake up call for me, definitely not what I wanted my future to bring.

One of the very first steps I took toward better health was giving up Sweet N' Low. I used to drink two 20-ounce coffees every day, one in the morning and one in the afternoon. Luckily, someone got it through my head that artificial sweeteners were bad for me, so I switched to sugar instead (the lesser of two evils). Sweet N' Low is actually saccharin in a packet, which was taken off the shelves for awhile when it was deemed unsafe for human consumption, but it is now readily available again for purchase.

You are probably also familiar with the other artificial sweeteners, NutraSweet or Equal (aspartame) and Splenda (sucralose) among others. The bottom line is that these artificial sweeteners are just that, artificial. There is nothing natural about them, they are chemical compounds and they are not in any way keeping you healthy (no matter what their marketing agents tell you). Artificial sweeteners can actually make you more hungry and also lower your metabolism. Read your labels through, because aspartame is found in over 6000 different food items on grocery shelves. Sugar is not a perfect choice, but in comparison to these choices, it was one step in the right direction for me.

Another change that I decided to make early on my healing path was suggested by Dr. Andrew Weil. He said, "Go on a news fast." At the time, I was a news (and TV) junkie. I watched the news every day, closing my night with the 10 o'clock news in bed. And I read the newspaper every single day as well. I did not realize how much the news was contributing to my stress levels. Taking a week off made such a significant difference in my state of being that I decided to continue that fast for some time. It was amazing to find how I could still get the news through connecting with others in my life, without needing to watch TV or read the papers. Today, I read in moderation and I feel well enough informed about important matters going on in the world today.

"Be the change you wish to see in the world."

~ Gandhi ~

CHAPTER 8

Going Free Range

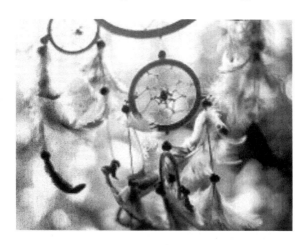

After taking blue green algae for 4 years, I was still coming home from work completely exhausted. Because my job wasn't overly stressful, I began looking at what I ate. I noted my eating habits throughout the day. I wasn't the healthiest eater. I was living to eat. The pleasure of taste and texture drove my food choices, rather than the benefit these foods had on my body. It wasn't hard to find the culprits that were draining my energy.

First, it started with my morning bagel (not the morning bagel)!! Yes, I still love bagels but they are no longer on my food plan. Bagels, especially large New York-style bagels, really do a number on the sugar levels in your body. Sure, they taste good, but they also spike the blood sugar and you may retain that happy good feeling for an hour or two before the crash comes. This fact is true for everyone, whether you are heavy or thin ~ it is basic body chemistry.

When your blood sugar crashes you will get tired and go looking for a pick-me-up, whether it's another simple carb or a cup of coffee to get you through the afternoon. My day was still full of sugar spikes throughout, up, down, up, down, up, down, until I was exhausted upon returning home with no energy to do anything except sit in front of the television and vegetate.

It was during this time that I was also educated on the truth of the meat industry and the fact of factory farming. John Robbins' book, *A Diet for a New America,* changed my mind about eating meat and chicken out at restaurants any longer, and I started buying organic free-range chicken products, grass-fed beef and bacon with no nitrates added. On top of that, I stopped visiting fast food restaurants as well. I never actually thought I could make that change since I had frequented them so often. But I was committed to better health and I knew on a very gut level (he he) that those establishments were not nourishing my body in any way.

These days, more and more information is being released about the processing of foods (if you still want to call it food) in these fast food restaurants. Have you heard about the pink slime that McDonald's uses in its burgers? If not, take a moment to research for that information, it is worth it.

Going through the pantry can be a daunting experience when you're not sure what you're looking for. One of the services my clients appreciate the most is my "Pantry Purge" service. It'll save you time getting on the right track! When you're ready, send me an e-mail with "Pantry Purge" in the subject line and we'll have a conversation.
trishbliss@me.com.

"When you are attracted to, and eat, fruits, occasionally a seed will be carried within you to a fertile ground."

~ David Wolfe ~

CHAPTER 9

Stepping Forward Into Health

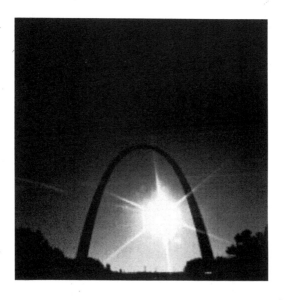

W hen I had left my corporate job at the insurance company to pursue a career in yoga, it was a big move in my life. To supplement my income in the beginning years, I worked at a local health food store and received a real education about whole foods, household toxins and the world of supplements. It had only been since 1996 that genetically modified organisms (GMOs) had started hitting the shelves of supermarkets in America, although there are still many people today who have not even heard of them.

I clearly remember the store's owner, Stephen, explaining to me that it had been proven that genetically modified foods actually genetically modify those who eat them! And it is true! GMOs have been proven to modify the DNA of the healthy bacteria that live in your gut, which can lead to a long list of maladies.[18]

If you Google GMOs, the first thing you will see at the top of the page will be GMO Benefits from Monstanto.com. Monsanto is the maker and distributor of these genetically modified foods and while I'm sure they believe they are helping humanity in some way, the fact is that over 25 countries around the globe have already outlawed the distribution of genetically modified foods.

---

[18] T.M Hartle, "Genetically Modified Organisms Inject DNA into Intestinal Bacteria," *Natural News* (June 24, 2011) *http://www.naturalnews.com/032800_GMOs_intestinal_bacteria.ht ml*

GMO animal studies have shown evidence of organ damage, gastrointestinal and immune disorders, as well as infertility and accelerated aging effects.[19] Human studies have also shown how GMO-soy can transfer into the DNA of bacteria inside of us and indeed genetically modify our bodies!

Since GMOs were introduced to the public, numerous health problems have increased including food allergies, autism, digestive illnesses among other dysfunctions. The American Public Health Association and the American Nurses Association are two of many medical organizations against the use of the genetically modified bovine growth hormone that is given to cows, because it has been linked to certain cancers.[20] GMO crops also cross-pollinate ~ so they can spread their seeds and contaminate nearby crops that are non-GMO or organic.

It is also important to note that Monsanto is the maker of Round-Up, a potent herbacide

---

[19] Jeffrey Smith, "10 Reasons to Avoid GMOs," *Institute for Responsible Technology* (August 25, 2011) *http://responsibletechnology.org/10-Reasons-to-Avoid-GMOs/*

[20] Jeffrey Smith, "Court Victory: Bovine Growth Hormone Labeling,"*Huffington Post Blog*, May 25, 2011 *http://www.huffingtonpost.com/jeffrey-smith/court-victory-bovine-grow_b_751009.html*

used on agricultural crops. They also make
Round-Up Ready Crops that are designed to
survive many applications of the Round-Up
(kind of scary). Round-Up itself has also been
linked with sterility, hormone disruption, birth
defects and cancer and is also outlawed in
some (wise) countries.[21]

There are also unfortunate close links with
the U.S. government and Monsanto. You
would easily be able to find more information
about how many former Monsanto employees
now work for the government. One such
person is Michael Taylor, who was both
Monsanto's attorney and their former vice
president. He is currently the U.S. Food Safety
Czar, which is a very strange title in my
opinion.

---

[21] Jeffrey Smith, "Damaging Effects of Roundup," Institute of
Responsible Technology,
http://responsibletechnology.org/docs/damaging-effects-of-roundup.pdf

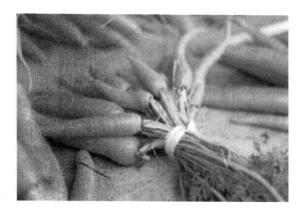

I remember the first bite of an organic vegetable that I ever tried ~ it was a carrot. And my very first thought was, "Maybe I don't actually like carrots after all." It was so carroty and I had never tasted a flavor quite so potent. I had become accustomed to bland tomatoes and tasteless carrots and I thought that was just the way they were supposed to taste.

Whenever I would eat a local (a.k.a. conventionally/pesticide grown) apple, my whole scalp would start tingling. However, that didn't happen when I ate an organic apple. Similarly, my sister became severely allergic to conventionally grown strawberries and would break out in hives all over her body. But coincidentally, she had no reaction when she consumed organic strawberries.

If you don't feel ready to fully go organic, at least you can avoid GMOs in your food purchases. By avoiding genetically modified foods, you contribute to the efforts to ban them by forcing them out of the food supply.

But how do you even know if something is genetically modified? Since there are still no current laws about correctly labeling genetically modified foods, the only way you can know if a food is clean is by looking for the package labels that state NON-GMO. Non-GMO companies want you to know that they are GMO-free, it is important to them! If you don't see such a label on a package, you can assume that it does contain genetically modified materials.

If you are looking at fruits and vegetables in the produce department of your local food store, they do in fact have specific labeling for them. Note that the conventionally grown produce have only 4 digits.

5 digits 9-xxxx Starting with 9 means ORGANIC
5 digits 8-xxxx Starting with an 8 means GMO
4 digits xxxx Conventionally grown,
**   may contain PESTICIDES**

Commonly known at the *Dirty Dozen*,[22] the following fruits and vegetables contain the highest amounts of pesticides, so if you are making choices, try to buy these produce items as organic whenever possible:

THE DIRTY DOZEN

1) Apples
2) Peaches
3) Nectarines
4) Strawberries
5) Grapes
6) Celery
7) Spinach
8) Sweet bell peppers
9) Cucumbers
10) Cherry Tomatoes
11) Imported Snap Peas
12) Potatoes

---

[22] EWG's 2015 Shopper's Guide to Pesticides in Produce, *http://www.ewg.org/foodnews/summary.php*

And now that you've learned the worst
foods to buy conventionally, also take note
of the best ones to buy conventionally,
they're called the *Clean 15*

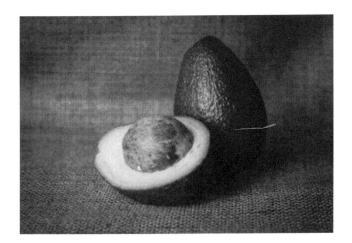

The Clean 15

1. *Avocados*
2. *Sweet Corn*
3. *Pineapples*
4. *Cabbage*
5. *Frozen Sweet Peas*
6. *Onions*
7. *Asparagus*
8. *Mangoes*
9. *Papayas*
10. *Kiwis*
11. *Eggplant*
12. *Grapefruit*
13. *Cantaloupe*
14. *Cauliflower*
15. *Sweet Potatoes*

*"The better you feed yourself, the stronger you will feel
and the bigger impact you will have on the world."*

~ Joshua Rosenthal ~

CHAPTER 10

Super Foods To The Rescue

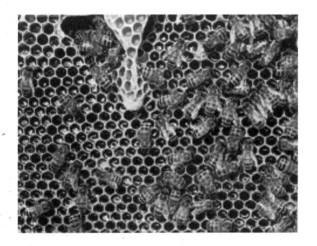

Super foods are food packed with a punch (in a good way)! They contain high amounts of nutrients in which the human body can readily absorb. You can integrate the following foods into your diet. I've introduced these items one by one by experimenting with them in my smoothies and soups and eggs.

Goji Berries contain 18 amino acids which include all 8 essential amino acids and have been used in Chinese medicine for over 5,000 years. They are known to help build strength in the body and assist with longevity as well.

Maca is an adaptogenic food, which means if you need energy it will help or if you need to calm down it will help. It contains almost 20 amino acids and 7 essential amino acids. It's said to help with strength, endurance and energy levels.

Blue Green Algae is the super food mentioned earlier in the book with which I had amazing results in turning my poor health around. Spirolina is another form of blue green algae and is also taken in tablet or capsule form to boost immunity.

Cacao is the raw form of chocolate and has among the highest antioxidants on the whole planet. In order for chocolate to be a health food, it must be at least 70% cacao, so read your labels to get the best!

Hemp products are high in protein and are one of the few plant-based sources of Omega 3 essential fatty acids. With its increased popularity, you can now find hemp seeds that you can add to soups, salads, eggs, and smoothies among other things. There are also other hemp protein products and hemp milk.

Sea Vegetables in essence are seaweed products. These include dulse, arame, hijiki, kelp, kombu and wakame. They can be added to soups, salads and stir fry. Nori is the seaweed wrapped around a sushi roll. Sea vegetables are said to remove heavy metals in the body and also to help detoxify the body of radioactive iodine. They may also support hormone health, including the thyroid and adrenal glands.

Bee products include honey (local is best), pollen and propolis. Raw honey, which is much thicker and tastier in my opinion, is rich in probiotics, minerals and enzymes. Pollen can be used in smoothies, too, as it contains nearly all the B vitamins and 21 essential amino acids which makes it a complete protein.[23]

---

[23] David Wolfe, "Superfoods: The Food and Medicine of the Future," (2009), Institute of Integrative Nutrition lecture 2015

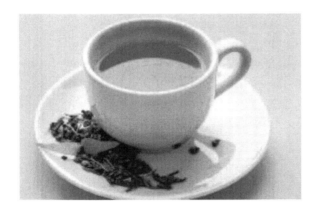

The Antioxidant Remedy ~
Antioxidants promote good health in the
body so remember to have a rainbow on
your plate to help fight oxidation!

Green Tea: Some consider green tea
the healthiest drink of the planet. It is full
of antioxidant properties that promote good
health in your body, from brain function to
cholesterol levels.

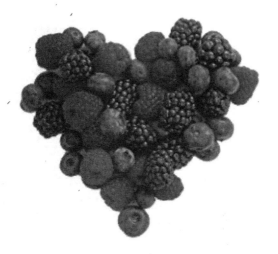

Blueberries are great for your eyes! I have fond memories of going over to the neighbor's house when I was growing up and feasting on their blueberry bush. It's best to eat things in season, but for me berries are the exception to that rule. All berries are good for you, but better for you without the pesticides, of course.

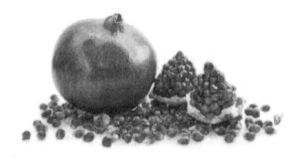

Pomegranates are known to be anti-inflammatory fruits. The seeds inside the fruit are edible and now you'll often find them in the stores already harvested for you. Pomegranates have an astringent and also a bitter quality that help to balance your body chemistry.

Acai is another super antioxidant fruit from Central and South America. You can find the powder form online or frozen in the health food store. It's another great addition to your smoothie!

Spinach needs no introduction, Popeye was onto something! Frozen spinach is better than canned, fresh is better than frozen. Spinach is full of phytonutrients and is thought to be one of the healthiest foods around.

Nuts & Seeds are best when they have been soaked overnight (or for 7-24 hours). You will be amazed how different a nut can taste! I have found them to be so much more filling as well so instead of eating 20, I want only 5 instead. Soaking your nuts and seeds makes them more digestible for your body and it removes inhibitors that naturally preserve the nut until water is present to begin its germination.

Interested in the best resources for these Super Foods? Send me an e-mail with "Super Foods" in the subject line for a list of the best places to get them and what to incorporate first. trishbliss@me.com.

"The more we pour the big machines, the fuel, the pesticides, the herbicides, the fertilizer and chemicals into farming, the more we knock out the mechanism that made it all work in the first place."

~ David R. Brower ~

CHAPTER 11

Inflammatory Foods

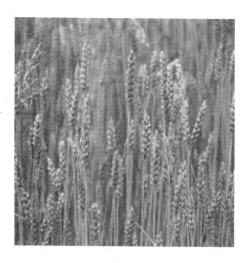

The first time I saw an acupuncturist she told me, "You have a bog living inside of you." Those were not exactly the words I wanted to hear. I had made such strides in my health by then, maintaining a consistent weight for about 5 years, I had opened a yoga studio and I felt like I had finally arrived at a good state of health. Then she suggested that I

give up all dairy products and I totally freaked
out (inside). Dairy products were my life line
as I was eating large amounts of cheese,
cottage cheese, half & half in my coffee,
butter, and of course, ice cream. How could I
live without it? I didn't think it was possible.
But I made the change. I gave up all forms of
(cow) dairy for a couple of years and I
adjusted surprisingly well. Things that I could
not bear to be without were replaced with
other things that were better for my health.

      Even though I had regained some health
and was not suffering from any obvious
symptoms, I was still dealing with cellular
inflammation in my body. There are certain
types of foods that cause inflammation in the
body including cow dairy products among
them. Sugar is another one. Some people have
sensitivity to these food items, which means
their body does not tolerate them and in turn, it
fights against them causing inflammation.

Top 10 Food Allergens

1. *Wheat/Gluten*
2. *Dairy*
3. *Corn*
4. *Eggs*
5. *Beef/Pork*
6. *Shellfish*
7. *Soy*
8. *Oranges*
9. *Peanuts*
10. *Refined Sugars*

Gluten is a food item that many people find they have a hard time processing. My gluten allergy just happened one day when my body said, "No more gluten!" It took me months to figure it out because I had never had any adverse reactions before. I got tested for gluten sensitivity at my naturopathic doctor, but it came up negative. Still, every time I ate it my digestion would be screwed up for a week. My body just did not want to tolerate it any longer. Gluten is a protein strain found in wheat, barley and rye and all their variations.

Obvious places to find it are in breads and cakes and cookies, but it also hides in many unusual places, so if you are sensitive be sure to make a habit of reading labels.

Some obscure places you may find gluten include bouillon cubes, canned soups, chocolate, flavored tofu, pickles, hotdogs, salad dressings, flavored chips, gravies, tamari and many condiments. Food manufacturers have taken to advertising their products as Gluten Free, so often times you can find that designation on the label.

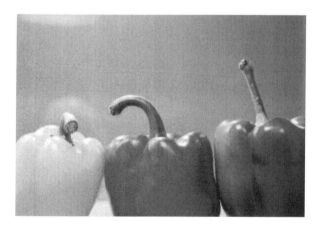

Nightshades are vegetables that actually grow at night. They have a great lore about their magic qualities but to some they cause inflammation in the body.

Nightshades include potatoes, tomatoes, eggplant, and all forms of peppers and spices made from peppers except for black pepper, which is exempt. Nightshades are not necessarily bad for you but you may want to avoid them if you have a compromised immune system or an autoimmune disease.[24] Nightshades have been linked with arthritis and joint pain but every person is different, so some find relief by avoiding them and others find no change whatsoever.

If you are suffering, it makes sense to experiment and take the necessary food items out of your diet for 3-4 weeks and when you add them back in, pay close attention to how you feel as a result.

---

[24] Elisha McFarland, "The Link Between Nightshades, Chronic Pain and Inflammation,"*GreenMedInfo,* April 21, 2013, *http://www.greenmedinfo.com/blog/link-between-nightshades-chronic-pain-and-inflammation*

*"You can't force a rosebud to blossom
by hitting it with a hammer."*

~ Rachel Naomi Remen, MD ~

CHAPTER 12

Feeding Your Body Well

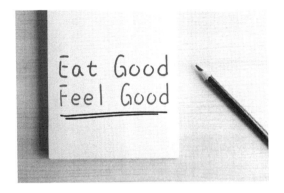

So in an ideal world, we would all subsist on whole fruits as our only sugar source. I have tried and tried for that to be my reality, but at some point or another I want more. So I began looking for recipes that were gluten free (and dairy free whenever possible) in which I could use alterative sugars. Some were really good, and some not so much.

I like going on recommendations from friends so I'm not wasting my time and money on something that is less than satisfying. But we live in good times and alternative recipes are available in plentitude. Things you want to avoid are cane juice sweetened or evaporated cane juice as these are simply regular refined sugar. There are supposedly 54 different names for sugar on packaging, so learn what you can and move in the right direction.

Here are some natural sugar options that have lower glycemic indexes (they won't make your blood sugar rise too quickly) and you can adapt into your lifestyle.

Stevia is an herb that is native to South America. It comes in both powered and liquid forms. If you use too much it can make your food taste bitter, but in the right amounts, it is the perfect way to fully enjoy the sweetness in your life since it contains no calories and has no glycemic index.

Coconut Sugar is also low on the glycemic index, meaning you won't get a buzz followed by a crash. You can replace coconut sugar for traditional sugar in all recipes, and although it is not as sweet as conventional sugar, it is satisfying.

Molasses maintains many of its nutritional benefits because of the way it is processed. Blackstrap molasses is a great source of both calcium and iron. I use it when I make homemade granola.

Pure Maple Syrup is another alternative you can use. It also has a lower rating on the glycemic index so it won't spike your sugar as quickly as white sugar. Be sure you are using pure maple syrup and not a product with any other ingredients on the label.

Supplementing Your Health

In an ideal world, we'd be getting all our supplements from our food, but unfortunately that is not the case these days. If you were eating a 100% local and organic diet that was completely well rounded, the odds would be in your favor. But the fact is that the soil conventional farmers use has been depleted of nutrients from overuse and pesticides. Below, are several supplements that can help you move in the direction of better health.

Probiotics are the first supplement I started taking after some years on the blue green algae. Probiotics are considered "good" bacteria because they keep your gut healthy. If your gut health is way off, be sure to purchase a high quality probiotic. Cheaper brands will not make it through your stomach acid properly to propagate in your intestines. You also want a probiotic with multiple varieties of bacteria strands.

You can also receive your probiotics through your food which is a more efficient way of populating the microbiota in your gut. Some of these are raw sauerkraut, kim chi, plain yogurt (goat yogurt can be an option for some), kefir, kombucha and miso among others.

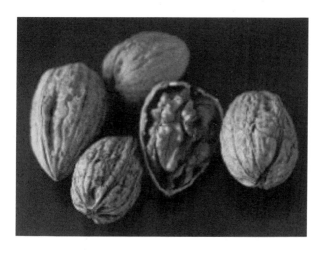

Omega Essential Fatty Acids have had their fanfare in the media as of late. Our bodies need these fatty acids for many functions from the building of healthy cells to maintenance of healthy brain and nerve function. They are very important since our bodies don't make them on their own, we must take them in through food or supplements.

Omega 3's are part of a broad group of fats labeled polyunsaturated fats. Common sources of omega 3's are salmon and flax seeds but less known are walnuts and sardines. Beef is also a high source of Omega 3's but only if it is grass-fed beef. Another common source is cod liver oil, but essential fatty acids can also be found in plant-based resources such as leafy green vegetables or other plant-based Omega 3 supplements.

Magnesium helps support your immune system, cleanse your gastro-intestinal tract and energize your whole body! It's also known to relieve occasional constipation and keep everything flowing smoothly throughout your digestive system. Magnesium can also aid your muscles and nerve work more effectively while controlling inflammation in the body. Because magnesium helps to metabolize carbohydrates after a meal, a magnesium deficiency in your body will put you at a greater risk of getting Type II diabetes.

Vitamin D is another important supplement to promote good health in your body. On the first few visits to my naturopath, she commented how it was truly a wellness visit. But we had blood work taken anyway and found I was quite deficient in Vitamin D. It seems this is very common, especially in New England. In the northern states, it is said we only get enough Vitamin D during the summer months and you have to wear no sunscreen in order to absorb it. It's a good idea to get your levels checked and follow the recommendations from a doctor or naturopath on how much you need to supplement.

Multi-Vitamins have long been touted as an essential part of a healthy diet. But every time I tried one, I would get shooting pains in my stomach shortly afterwards. This was very unusual for me, since I never have any stomach problems. It was also quite disappointing, as I had just spent mucho bucks on another bottle of useless pills. But I have found a wonderful multi-vitamin that is coated in aloe so it does not disrupt my belly at all. The other important thing to note in a multi-vitamin is the color of the water after you use the toilet. When the color is a neon-yellow it means that most of the nutrients have passed out of you. Give your body what it needs and you will feel the results of your efforts.

There are many other supplements on the market and each individual has to research and find out what their body needs. I believe it is best to work with a consultant to determine your needs and then find the right supplements to give your body a boost in the direction of greater health. Good supplements are expensive but well worth the money.

In my opinion, it is better to buy high quality supplements and receive a benefit from them, than buying a grocery store brand (which are still pricey) whose quality is low and often ineffective. You may not need to take certain supplements forever, just until your body starts working properly on its own again.

*Atha yoga anushasanam : Now, the
teachings of yoga.*

~ Yoga Sutra 1.1 ~

CHAPTER 13

Look Out For The Chemicals

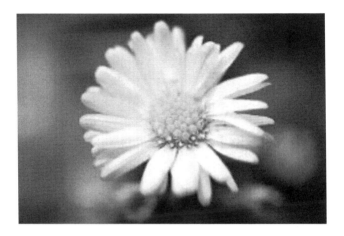

It was still some years after my introduction to yoga that I learned about the hazards of using anti-bacterial products. As it was explained to me, when you use those products, they are actually doing your immune system's job for it and the result is weakened immunity.

You actually want your immune system to do its good work for you as it gets exercised that way and learns to combat germs in a new way. Each time you get a cold or the flu, your immune system is strengthened. Being too clean is actually bad for your health and our sterile lifestyles have compromised our own healing capabilities.

By this time you have probably deduced that health is more than just what you eat. There are everyday activities that either support or harm your body's vitality. My time working at the local health food store taught me so much about healthy living and why germs are sometimes good for you! For instance, the Federal Drug Administration has reported that anti-bacterial soaps were ineffective and could indeed be harming you!

According to a Smithsonian magazine article[25], the top reasons not to use anti-bacterial soaps are as follows:

1. They are not more effective than conventional soap and water.

---

[25] Joseph Stromberg, "Five Reasons Why You Should Probably Stop Using Antibacterial Soap," *Smithsonian.com*, January 3, 2014, *http://www.smithsonianmag.com/science-nature/five-reasons-why-you-should-probably-stop-using-antibacterial-soap-180948078/?no-ist*

2. *Anti-bacterial soaps have the potential to create antibiotic-resistant bacteria.*
3. *They could act as endocrine disruptors and interfere with thyroid regulation.*
4. *They could lead to other problems including allergies.*
5. *They are bad for the environment.*

There are also alcohol-based products that kills bacteria but don't really clean your hands. A good scrub (try some homemade soap before it's outlawed) for 30 seconds will do the trick.

Another step that I took towards better health was to change from conventional shampoo and conditioner products to ones that are all natural. Try reading the back of your shampoo bottle and see how many words you can actually recognize. Chemicals in shampoos, detergents, carpeting and other consumer products have never been thoroughly tested. There are health concerns all around. Prescription medications and pesticides have to go through vigorous studies before they are released for human consumption and yet thousands upon thousands of chemicals are introduced into our environment (home and otherwise) without any authorization whatsoever.

"Unlike pharmaceuticals or pesticides, industrial chemicals do not have to be tested before they are put on the market. Under the law regulating chemicals, producers are only rarely required to provide the federal government with the information necessary to assess safety."[26]

Using all natural body lotions, hand creams and household products can indeed improve your health. As mentioned in Urbina's 2013 *New York* Times article (see footnote below), there are over 85,000 chemicals added into consumer products and only a small percentage of those have been safety-tested. Even for the few that have been tested, they are not tested in conjunction with other chemicals. So whereas one chemical could be deemed "safe," they don't really know how it reacts with any other chemical.

Another important ingredient to look out for is aluminum. Many years ago I made the change to natural deodorant and gave up the

---

[26] Ian Urbina, "Think Those Chemicals Have Been Tested?" *New York Times*, April 13, 2013

antiperspirant because most (if not all) of them contain aluminum. Aluminum has been linked to breast cancer among other diseases so it's a good idea to stop putting it underneath your arms every day.[27] Manufacturers may say a product contains no harmful aluminums but know that there is no such thing as beneficial aluminums. I also got rid of my aluminum cookware and stopped using Teflon pans. Teflon is relatively safe as long as it never gets scratched. If it does get scratched, however, harmful chemicals can leak into your food while you are cooking so cast iron and stainless steel are the better options for cookware. Besides deodorant and cookware, you can also look for aluminum in some baking powders, food coloring such as Yellow #5 and some vaccines.

Essential oils are a chemical-free alternative to the otherwise harsh products on the market. Interested in learning more about essential oils? Send me an e-mail with "Essential Oils" in the subject line and I'll send you some fun things to incorporate that are simple to use. trishbliss@me.com.

---

[27] Michelle Goldstein, "New Research Links Aluminum to Breast Cancer," *Natural News* (September 27, 2013) *http://www.naturalnews.com/042235_aluminum_breast_cancer_en vironmental_toxins.html*

"Beautify your thoughts.
Thoughts are the headwaters of
action, life and manifestation."

~ David Wolfe ~

CHAPTER 14

Remedies For An Ailing Body

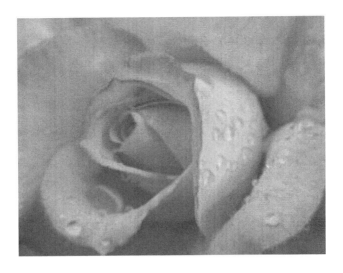

When I was young, I loved playing tag with the neighborhood kids and running as fast as I could so my heart was pounding in my head when I reached home base. And I loved jump rope, too, and I was a wiz at double-dutch jump rope when I was in elementary school! But then my food coma set in, it must have been around junior high time when I stopped moving and started vegetating in front of the television set. I stopped playing with the neighborhood children and never even wanted to go outside anymore. We were not a family to exercise together, so it was not surprising that I fell into the pit of inertia.

I joined softball and soccer when I entered high school so it would look good on my college resumes. It took until my senior year in high school before the soccer coach saw how fast I could actually run and put me on the front lines as a forward on the playing field. I've never been a distant runner, but I do love sprinting ~ the short & sweet bursts of energy leave me feeling alive!!

When determining what exercise you LOVE, it is good to remember back to your youth and think about what you enjoyed doing back then. There is a good chance you will still like that activity or something similar to it. I would never describe myself as a star athlete by any means, but I have found ways to move my body that feel good to me.

I was in the worst shape of my life when I was 25-years-old. I was about 50 pounds overweight and miserable in all aspects of the word. I did not know what I wanted to do as a career in life and I was lost as to how to find happiness. I had a terrible diet at the time, even though ironically, I had been a vegetarian

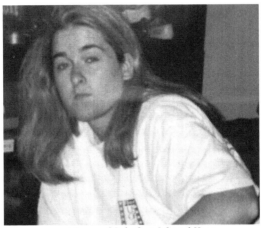

Me, age 25, before I found Yoga

for 3 years. When I first started going to the gym, I would come out of a step aerobics class with my face crimson-colored, looking like I was going to have a heart attack at any moment. At the time, I didn't like the idea of exercising at all, but I did love step aerobics! Of course, after a few years my knees weren't too happy with me, but I knew that I must find activity that I liked in order to do it regularly.

In those days I would only exercise in spring and summer and I would literally hibernate all fall and winter. That is until I started taking yoga classes one winter ~ that was definitely a game-changer for me! Yoga was different from any other type of exercise I had ever tried and I was hooked from the very first class.

I liked all the different kinds of postures but especially enjoyed the relaxation at the end of the class! Like many students, I lived for Savasana (relaxation pose). All of the effort was worth it, as long as I could lie down and be still for those few minutes at the end of the practice. It was the icing on the cake for me long before I knew the deep healing capacity of that posture. They say if you can only do one yoga posture a day, let it be Savasana.

You can think of Savasana as a posture of conscious relaxation. Lie on your back (usually on the floor) with your palms turned up at your sides and your eyes closed.

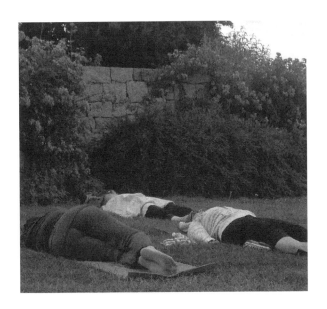

But staying awake while lying in a relaxed position is where the real healing happens. Your parasympathetic nervous system is activated in that state, which instills relaxation in your body. When you learn to deeply relax yourself (without falling asleep) there is great healing benefit for your whole body.

"Your task is not to seek for love, but merely to seek and find all the barriers within yourself that you have built."

~ Rumi ~

CHAPTER 15

The Practice of Yoga Begins

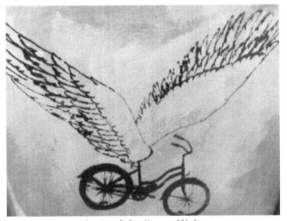

Artwork by Susan Hickman

Yoga had such a powerful impact on my life that I decided to become a teacher myself in order to share the wonderful benefits I had received through the practice. At the time, I was working in the insurance industry in Hartford, CT, and had saved all my vacation days for a year so that I could take a full month off to take the teacher training. My friends at work had other ideas though and they secured me in a conference room one afternoon to have a sort of intervention. "Don't come back," they said. "If you come back, you'll never leave," and they said this out of love. "We can't leave, but you can!" So, I took the leap into my career in yoga and haven't regretted it for a moment. Although we've mostly lost touch since then, those friends had a mighty powerful effect upon the course of my life.

After spending a month at yoga teacher training, I arrived back home at the end of March. It was a warm spring that year and when I got on my bike for my maiden ride of the year, something wonderful had happened...instead of breathing heavy and having all my leg muscles screaming at me, the intense month of yoga practice had completely changed my body! For the first time in my life, I actually felt like I was in shape! I felt good in my body, both strong and limber.

And things have gotten even better for me in that category even as I have aged since then. Yoga has an amazing effect on the body and the mind. And yes, there are many types of yoga available today so it is important to find a style of yoga and a teacher to whom you feel connected in order to get the most out of the practice. I hear so many people say, "I tried yoga once." And although, it is true that yoga is not for everyone, I believe more likely it is because they did not find the right teacher or a style of yoga with which they could resonate.

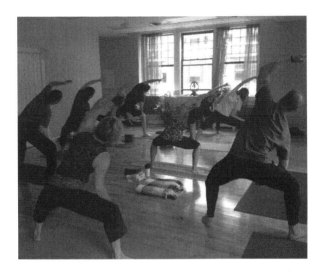

Through my yoga practice, I was opened up to other types of exercise as well. It is so very important to find some way to move your body that you enjoy Some people like the machines at the gym. Some like doing their own thing, while others prefer group activities (like yoga or spinning classes). I have found that I like outdoor activities more than indoor. I loved roller skating when I was young, and now I have a cool pair of rollerblades to help get myself moving. But I am most happy when taking a hike in the woods or along the beach.

Another great tip I've learned through the years is the benefit of breathing through your nose while exercising. Dr. John Douillard's book *Body, Mind, Sport* goes into great details about the science behind the theory. But the long and short of it is that mouth-breathing creates a fight-or-flight reaction in the nervous system. Breathing in and out of your nose will keep you calm while you exercise.

If you have a regular exercise routine and start this practice, you will most likely find you have to do a little less for a while until you adjust. But when you continue the practice, you'll find that you will go well beyond your previous workout capacity ~ many professional athletes have found this to be true. You tap into "the zone" or your superhuman capacity because you are calm and centered while your body is moving at warp speed (or even just walking down the road).

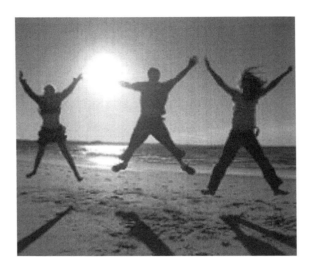

Nobody can tell you what is best for you, as we each need to take on that path of self-discovery. Be curious and try new ways of moving your body. Do you love dancing (or did you love it once)? Put on some good music and dance yourself into shape! Or try one push-up with your knees on the floor and build up from there. To get the healthiest results, it is best to be consistent with your exercise. Instead of doing an hour walk once a week, it is better to try for 15 minutes a day.

Cross training is working different muscles groups through different activities such as walking one day and biking on another. If you only stay with one activity or one sequence of poses in yoga, you will only be working certain muscles instead of all of them. You want to be strong and flexible all over.

If you prefer inspiration and support in a group setting, Blissworks Yoga and Healing Arts offer a variety of class levels and packages to meet you where you are. http://blissworksyoga.org/

"Become the person who, when you walk in a room everyone is blessed."

~ Tosha Silver ~

CHAPTER 16

Meditation Is Exercise For The Mind

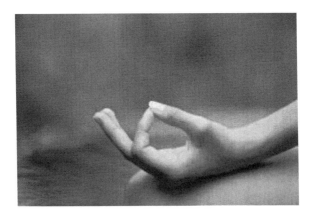

Because I've been practicing yoga for so long now, people assume that I took to it quite easily. But my mind has been just as crazy as everyone else's as it the nature of the mind is to move. So, while we want to get the body moving in order to be healthy, we actually want the mind to slow down for better health. Many misunderstand meditation because they say, "I can't slow down my mind," or "my mind never stops." Well, that awareness is the start of your meditation practice. There are innumerable ways to practice meditation, and it is important to find the method that works best for you.

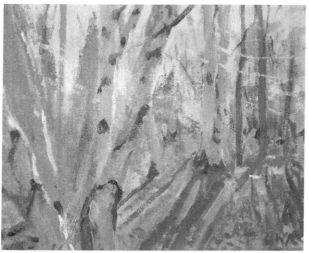

Artwork by Charles W. Reyburn

A good friend of mine paints as his meditation. His is an open-eye meditation, observing the world around himself while focusing his attention on color, shape and perspective. The practice of concentration sometimes draws him into an altered state that he refers to as "non-verbal." He has mastered the practice of standing still in one place and looking closely at nature. He has even surprised a group of deer going through the forest because the depth of his own inner stillness. You don't have to start painting in order to find your inner stillness since there are endless ways to cultivate that for yourself. Some people use a walk as their meditation, a way to get some time on their own. As a yoga teacher, I am drawn to seated meditation.

The first step I teach in mediation practice is the art of sitting still. If you can remain still in your practice (especially the first three minutes), you will receive the greatest benefit. If you are new to a sitting practice, please begin with a 5 minutes. Commit to sitting still for 5 minutes a day for 40 days and you will notice a significant change in your life! Be sure to set a timer so you don't have to be concerned about the time. Just sit as still as possible and let your mind move any way it wants to move. You can sit in a chair or on a cushion on the floor, just be sure you are in a comfortable position.

The second step is to create a point of focus or a place of concentration for your practice. The simplest one is to use your breath as the focal point. Become aware of a place in your body where you notice your breath and allow yourself to focus on that sensation. Then whenever your mind wanders (and you realize your minding is wandering), bring your awareness back to that place of sensation.

Your mind can wander a million times, as it is the nature of the mind of wander. But as many times as you notice your mind wandering, that many times you can bring it back to your point of focus. Meditation is a practice of concentration. You can also add in a mantra or an affirmation to repeat silently to yourself. I always like saying *I am healed and whole.* Another one that I repeat regularly is, *I love my life!* Repeat these phrases to yourself regularly and see what shifts in your life.

Meditation has been proved scientifically to improve health.[28] It has been shown to relieve stress, anxiety, fatigue, help adjust moods and enhance sleep. There has also been evidence that shows meditation can lower blood pressure as well as improve the symptoms of menopause.

Breathing Your Way to Better Health

Further into my yoga practice I started daily breath work exercises. In yoga, we refer to this practice as pranayama and it is a way to learn to control your own life force energy.

Here are some breath exercises you can try.

---

[28] Susan Kuchinskas, "Meditation Heals Body and Mind," *WebMD Magazine, http://www.webmd.com/mental-health/features/meditation-heals-body-and-mind*

Dirgha Pranayama

This breathing technique is also called the yogic 3-part breath and it teaches you to expand to your full lung capacity. You can do this exercise either sitting or lying down, but whatever position you choose, start by placing your hands on your low belly area and breathe into your fingertips there. This is the first part of the 3-part breath and it teaches you to first breathe into the lower lobes of your lungs. As the lower lobes expand it causes your diaphragm to contract and press the organs of your abdomen out and into your hands. Do a couple rounds of breath here before moving to the next level.

Part two of the Dirgha pranayama also starts by inflating the low lobes of the lungs and then breathing into your side ribs. Place your hands on the sides of your rib cage so you can feel your lung expand into your own touch there. Breathe into the "belly" and then into the side ribs and then watch the ribs relax and the belly relax as your breath empties. The third part of the breath has your hands touching your collarbones at the top of your chest area. Just like filling a glass of water, you breathe into the bottom of your lungs and

then the middle (ribcage) and then sip in a last
bit of breath to lift into your fingertips at the
top of your chest. Find the place where you are
totally full and then slowly watch the breath
empty back out again. You fill from bottom to
top and empty from top to bottom. This
breathing practice takes a lot of concentration,
but it will teach you to slow down your
breathing and bring you into a state of
relaxation. It also helps your expand your
capacity of breath, which of course, has many
benefits as well. Start by practicing the Dirgha
pranayama for 5 minutes daily.

Ujjayi Pranayama

Ujjayi is translated as the Victorious Breath
and it is victorious indeed! This breathing
practice refines and lengthens your breathing
capacity as well as having a calming effect on
the mind. It calms the mind because it gives it
something on which it can pay attention, but it
is also from the soothing sound that you create
while practicing the breathing exercise.

The best way to learn this technique is to
take a deep inhalation through your nose and
release your breath through open lips, making
a soft haaaaaa sound. Do that a few times to
practice and then on one of your exhalations,

start through open lips and halfway through touch your lips together. If you did that, you should hear a soft sound in the back of your throat, this is the sound of Ujjayi. You can continue that way, or to go to the next level by keeping the muscles of your throat constricted as you continue your breath in and out of your nose. Be sure the sound remains in your throat as it is not a nasal sound. Contracting your throat muscles and slightly narrowing your breath passageway creates the sound of Ujjayi. Try 3-5 minutes of this breath exercise.

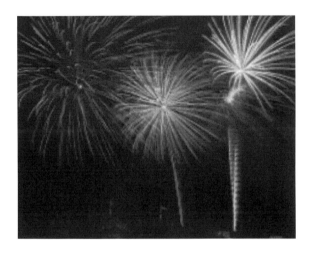

Kapalabhati Pranayama

This breathing exercise is more advanced, but it does help to cleanse the body of toxins. Because it is a more vigorous technique, it does have some precautions. Pregnant women should not practice this technique, nor should you practice if you have un-medicated high blood pressure, a detached retina or glaucoma. Other contraindications are recent surgery and injury or inflammation in the abdominal or thoracic region. Please call in the advice of a medical doctor or experienced yoga instructor if you are unsure.

The emphasis of this technique is on the rapid expulsion of breath on the exhalation. The inhalation should be passive and it will just happen naturally. Put your attention on the exhalation and the rapid pumping of air out of the body by contracting the diaphragm and know that your inhalation will take care of itself.

Start by taking a few deep and relaxing breaths. Then take a nice long inhalation and release a sharp short forceful exhalation through your nose. You can repeat this rapid expulsion several times slowly, concentrating on the forceful exhalation and allowing your inhalation to come naturally and without effort. You can start with 10 expulsions and then return to your normal breathing pattern.

If you find you are short of breath or feel

light-headed, slow down your efforts or stop all together. Kapalabhati is often translated as the "skull-polishing" breath and it is known to help clean and purify your nasal passages. It also shifts the cerebral spinal fluid by changing the rhythm of your normal respiration thus creating a massaging effect on your brain and enlivening every cell around the entire skull!

If you prefer guidance when doing breathing exercises, here's a CD to get you going: http://bit.ly/1Ra6AQb

"It does not matter how slowly you go as long as you do not stop."

~ Confucius ~

CHAPTER 17

Yoga Cleansing Practices

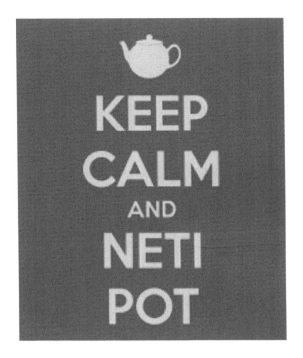

There are other cleansing practices that I have learned through yoga that help aid the body in its healing. I learned about the neti pot from very first yoga teacher back in 1995. It is used for nasal irrigation to rinse mucus and debris from your nasal passages and is very helpful for people prone to allergies or sinus infections but can be useful even if that is not the case for you.

It is recommended to use distilled warm water in your neti pot, but I have always used tap water myself. The most important part of this practice is to be sure the water is not too hot nor too cold as your sinuses can become very irritated by the wrong temperature. Warm water is good and you should be able to hold your finger in the water without any discomfort.

Use sea salt rather than an iodized salt variety though, and you will need ¼ teaspoon per side. Insert the tip of the neti pot into one nostril and tip your head to the side it will drain from. The water travels up one side and empties through the opposite nostril. When you are done one side, blow your nose and then repeat the same procedure on the other nostril. There have been cases of people supposedly using contaminated water and dying, so use sterilized or distilled water if you are concerned.

Oil pulling is also an amazing way to promote health in your body. You probably know the mouth can accumulate all types of harmful bacteria so oil pulling is one remedy to rid your body of them daily. It consists of using a small amount of organic oil (coconut, almond or sesame) and swishing it in your mouth for 10-20 minutes. Some recommend using a tablespoon of oil but I find that the swishing causes too much saliva to be released and I end up with too much liquid in my mouth, so I do about 1-2 teaspoons. Move it through your teeth and all around your mouth.

This is an easy practice to do when you are getting ready in the morning (and do not need to talk to anyone for a few minutes). I have also done the practice while taking a shower to save time. This practice is great for oral hygiene, preventing cavities, helping gingivitis and also pulling toxins from your sinus cavities. It has also whitened my teeth! When you have done your swishing, be sure to spit the discarded oil (and white foam) into the toilet or garbage bag. Do not spit into your sink as it is truly toxic by the time you are done and you do not want to spread the bacteria any further. Brush your teeth after you have completed the oil pulling practice.

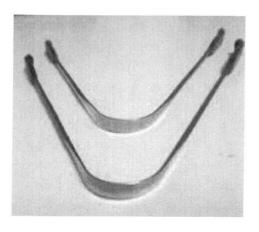

Another useful tool to help cleanse your body daily is a metal tongue scraper. This is a simple technique that helps to promote both oral and digestive health. Since your entire body is mapped on your tongue (just as it is on your hands, feet and ears), by gently stimulating your tongue in the morning it is also stimulating all your internal organs. This practice also helps to clear bacteria and toxins and enhance your taste buds. Because digestion begins with your sense of taste, this practice also aids in healthy digestion. It is important not to use a plastic tongue scraper as bacteria can accumulate on the plastic material. I use stainless steel, but any type of metal scraper is appropriate. To use the tongue scraper, hold it with both hands and place the rounded edge on the back of your tongue. Gently scrape to the front of the tongue between 5 and 15 times, rinsing it off between rounds if there is any accumulation on the scraper. If you tend to gag, either do not go so far back on your tongue or try a gentler stroke. This should be a daily practice for optimal health.

One more practice that I have taken to over the years is to alternate between hot and cold in the shower. I do this practice at the end of my shower, and honestly it does take a strong amount of willpower. After I have completed my ablutions, I turn the water to cold and once it switches over, I count to 10 while it hits the crown of my head. Then I turn it back to hot and count to 10 again and repeat this practice three times, ending on the cold cycle (although some recommend up to 7 cycles).

This therapy is extremely invigorating for your circulation system and to promote overall health and wellbeing. The reason it works is because when the body's outside temperature is hot, the flow of circulation goes out to the skin and when the body is subjected to cold, the flow of circulation moves to the internal organs. Thus, alternating between cold and hot moves the circulation in and out respectively and therefore helps to detoxify the body and also move nutrients to all parts of the body.

Consider changing your attitude about eating. Recognize it as a sacred ritual that deserves your attention. Bring consciousness into your eating habits and begin to notice your attitude and behaviors around food.

Mindful eating techniques:
- ○ *Give thanks! Show appreciation for your food and all the people who helped get the food to your plate. You can do this silently or aloud, but take a moment of pause before you start to eat.*
- ○ *Use smaller plates to control your portion and still feel like you're getting a full amount.*
- ○ *Put your fork/soup spoon/chopsticks down between bites and chew thoroughly. I have a habit of eating fast, and I know I'm not alone in that. When you eat quickly your body does not have time to process the amount of food you are eating, so there can be a tendency to overeat.*

- *Eat without distracting yourself. Avoid being on the computer or reading a book while you are eating. Instead, listen to some relaxing music that is conducive to good digestion.*
- *It is fine to engage in positive conversation while having a meal with someone but beware of highly fueled topics that bring up strong emotions when you eat. Your feelings have a direct effect on how your food is absorbed (or not absorbed) properly.*
- *Affirm your body and pay attention to when you are feeling full. I spent so many years eating past the point of satiation, so in order to change I had to pay strict attention to this detail. Generally, I find one moderate-sized plate is enough for me, no seconds.*

"Beware of creating your own stress."

~Howard Murad ~

CHAPTER 18

Food As An Addiction

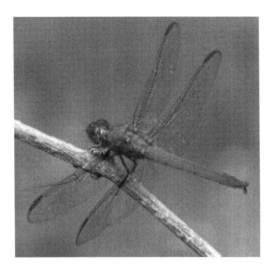

The first person to whom I admitted that I had a problem with food was my older sister. When I was 15 years old, she came home to tell me she had joined a support group for compulsive overeating. She had a list of 15 questions that determined if you were a compulsive eater and I passed with flying colors! I specifically remember saying, "Yeah, well, I don't care! I'm not giving up sugar!" It took me 15 more years before I was miserable enough to make a change. Having support around your food issues is essential in healing them. If you are isolated or alone, or feel like people in your family and life are unsupportive of you making a positive change for yourself, please seek out the company of others who understand what you are going through. They are out there waiting to meet you.

I have many friends now that I can call upon in my time of need. When I am feeling overwhelmed in life or down on myself for something or other, I make phone calls to seek the support I need. These people will not give me advice, instead they are all capable of holding space and listening to me. My friends recognize my ability to intelligently figure out my own life. They do not need to tell me what to do, but they may need to listen to me rant or cry, depending upon the day.

In those 15 years of growing up to adulthood, I was not happy. Most people did not recognize my unhappiness because I would always smile and be as pleasant as possible. But I was in a great deal of emotional pain. To the outside world I seemed like a happy girl but those who were close to me witnessed the level of misery to which I had sunk. It's hard to explain how emotional pain can build through the years. I was always looking for a miracle cure, one that would pop me into another body or another life where everything was glorious all the time.

In retrospect, I can see that the level of my unhappiness was directly linked to my wishing that my life (or more specifically, my body) could be different. I wanted different genetics and wished I had a different shaped body. I wished my skin wasn't quite so opaque. I felt like life had given me the rough end of the stick. And honestly, the only thing that made me "happy" during that time in my life was food.

I remember my boyfriend in college asking me if I loved him more than ice cream. I just laughed and told him not to ask questions if he didn't want to hear the answers. Ice cream was my love at the time and I didn't want anyone getting in the way of our good time together.

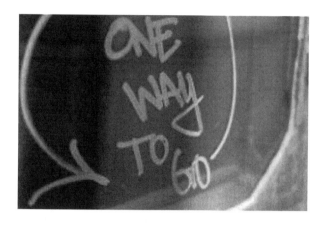

At the very beginning of my freshman year at college, my roommate and I were studying for our chemistry exam in the library. It was 11:30 PM and she suggested we head across campus for an ice cream. I was immediately on that plan and packed up my books and started racing down the stairs.

The ice cream place closed at midnight, so we would have to make good time walking across campus to get there. In the lobby, she saw her boyfriend and started talking. With great urgency, I told her we didn't have time to talk and as I was saying my good-byes I began to walk backwards at a good pace.

When I quickly turned around, I ran smack into a 40-foot bronze statue with my head, making a very loud BONG sound that resonated throughout the lobby as the narrow statue teetered on its base. The whole lobby went silent for a moment and then burst into laughter! I had fallen down with a giant egg on my forehead from hitting the artwork with such force. Needless to say, we didn't make it to the ice cream shop that night. I always think back at that being my very first wake-up call from the Universe.

So after so many years, why can't I stop eating things that I know are not good for me? This is a two-fold question for me. Firstly, I believe I am still sorting out the microbiome in my gut. Unfortunately, when things are out of whack in the gut and there is an overgrowth of yeast, it does send signals to the brain wanting more of what it wants. To some degree, I believe this is the root of all cravings.

Secondly, I am still learning to reprogram my brain from a lifetime of habitual behaviors. I have really come leaps and bounds in my recovery. Change does not happen overnight but with the right support system, we can all move in the direction of better living ourselves.

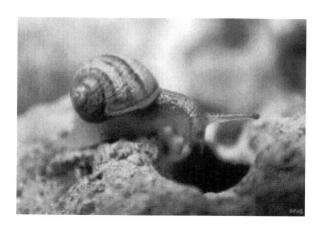

If I'd not made changes in my life, I might not be alive today. If I'd remained stagnant, I may still be alive but I'd certainly not be living and loving my life as I do now. And yet, I still start over every single day and sometimes I have begun again halfway through the day.

What I have learned is putting off the start until Monday or the New Year never really works. When I have promised myself to begin on a set date or after the weekend, I have found that it never sticks. The only time I have found peace is starting in the moment that I recognize I have gone astray, no matter what time of day it is and no matter what day of the week it is, I begin there.

One time I was flying to Florida for vacation and having dreams of this particularly amazing dessert I had had there before. The book I was reading was speaking about putting off the start date of your change until after you get the promotion or after you come back from the vacation. It was one of those moments when all the bells and whistles went off in my head and I recognized my long history of procrastination.

As painful as it was, I decided that moment not to have any sugar on vacation, including that one dessert about which I was dreaming. It didn't help that my friend on vacation decided to order the said dessert anyhow, but miraculously I did not squirm or cave at the temptation.

Because I have started over so many times, I have also found that I don't stray quite as far from my goals as I used to in the past. My periods off my plan are still there sometimes, but I don't dive so deep into the hole of depravity. I keep moving in the direction of my intentions and just like a meditation, no matter how many times I may lose my way, I have a focal point to return to and redirect my actions. These days I seriously wonder if I will ever "get there," meaning my ideal body weight or feeling totally content with myself as I am. But I am on for the ride, as this living thing is a process of growth.

I am clear about how I want to relate to myself and my world, so I will keep on moving in the direction of my intentions, throughout all the days of my life! I spent so many years deep in misery that I got quite tired of it. I found a new way of relating to myself, one that does not need to be so painful. And while I still have some bad days, for the most part my inner world does indeed reflect my outer world these days. I no longer have to put on one face for the world and another for my close friends and family.

Another lesson for me happened one day when I was griping that nobody ever smiled around me. It took me a moment to realize that I was the one never smiling. So, I started an exercise of consciously smiling at everyone I met. Because of the place I was at, I used to get upset if I smiled and someone didn't return the smile to me. Then I grew out of that and was able to freely offer smiles without expecting anything in return. And guess what, I felt better because of it. Smiling works to improve your mood and outlook on life, try it out!

Because I have been willing to face up against the uncomfortable parts of my being, I have seen more and more glimpses of the truth of who I am (and who you are as well). All of this life is temporary and I have decided that I want to make the most of it while I'm here. There is no use in wishing I were different than I am in any given moment, but I will continue to strive to be more loving and compassionate both to myself and those I meet in life as well.

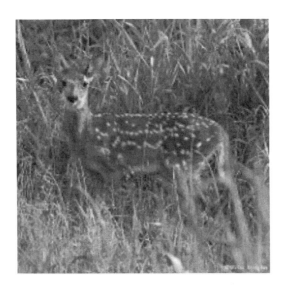

Learning to be gentle with myself through this process is my greatest learning and patience is one of my life-long lessons. It's funny how compassionate and loving I can be towards others who are in pain, but with myself, I'm still rather fierce.

I realize that healing doesn't happen overnight. I've been moving in the direction of my intention for many years now and I will continue moving in that direction and refining myself along the way.

The yoga philosophy that I teach from recognizes that we are all individual aspects of the one Divine energy that moves through all of life. A long time ago, I got stuck in my pain and somehow told myself that that was the way it was for me.

Repositioning my perspective and allowing self-awareness to unfold helps me to see my life experiences from a higher viewpoint. When I think I "should" be in a different (more evolved) place than I am currently in, I have the opportunity to step back and see the lesson that is in front of me. It gives me the chance to realize that everything is in Divine and perfect order, nothing needs to be different, not me, not you.

We're all just as we're supposed to be and yet there is a lesson in every single moment of life if we pay close enough attention.

"Your body is a temple, but only if you treat it as one."

~ Astrid Alauda ~

CHAPTER 19

Fall In LOVE With The Art Of Cooking

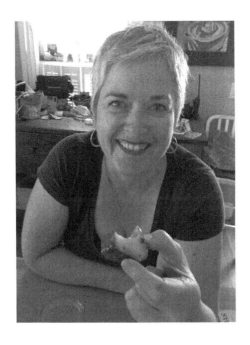

I grew up on canned and frozen food. Opening a can of Spagetti O's with Meatballs and heating it up on the stove was the extent of my cooking skills. Later I turned to the microwave that allowed less dishes to wash at the end of the meal.

When I did start cooking in my 20's my partner at the time did not like anything I cooked, so I stopped trying. Then when I was single for 7 years, I often ate out at restaurants or got take out instead of cooking for myself. It always felt like such a drag to come up with ideas of what to cook or to get myself to the grocery store to buy the required ingredients. Yet although I always knew I wanted more nourishing home-cooked meals, I could not get myself there for many years.

Now things have changed so much that I am often unsatisfied with food that I get out at restaurants. It's hard to find wholesome healthy food in most restaurants although there are a few around my area that never disappoint.

All of the years of accumulating healthy recipes have finally caught up to me. When I entered my health coach school, I realized that I have made significant changes in the types of good food I choose to eat these days. Even though I've been teaching yoga since the year 2000, I am not a vegetarian. I tried it out for 3 years but actually gained a considerable amount of weight because I ate a whole lot of pasta and bread and sugar while trying to avoid meat.

I believe there is a right diet for every individual and in order to find out what is right, we have to experiment with different ways of eating. Here are some recipes that will excite your taste buds and inspire you to try something new. All are both vegetarian and gluten free.

If you have some great recipes to share, let me know & I'll be happy to try them out!

Here's to delicious, healthy food that is simple to prepare!

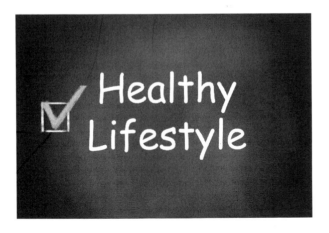

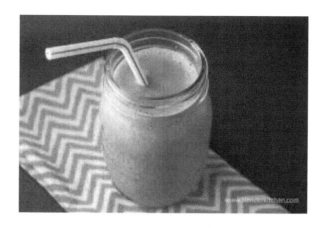

~ *Green Smoothie for Anti-Inflammation* ~

A Handful of Spinach
2 Kale Leaves
1 Leaf Collard Greens
½ Ripe Pear
½ Tart Apple
1 Small Chunk Ginger
1 Cup Water

Place all ingredients in a high-powered blender and process until smooth.

~ *My Favorite Green Juice* ~

2 Kale Leaves
2 Medium Carrots
½ Apple
1 Small to Medium Chunk Ginger

Process all ingredients through a juicer and enjoy!

~ *Homemade Granola* ~

4 Cups Gluten Free Oats
2/3 Cup Coconut
½ Cup Sunflower Seeds
1/3 Cup Almonds
1/8 Cup Flax Seeds
1 tsp. Cinnamon
Optional: Sesame Seeds, Pumpkin Seeds, other Nuts.
Preheat oven to 250 degrees. Mix above ingredients together in a large bowl.
In a small pan on the stove heat 1/3 Cup Molasses, 1/3 Cup Honey, 1/3 Cup Water, 2 Tbsp. Coconut Oil, splash of pure vanilla extract and bring to a boil. Pour over above mixture and cook until oats are lightly toasted.
Optional: Add raisins or dried cranberries after mixture has cooled.

~ *Butternut Squash Soup* ~

1 Butternut Squash
1 Tbsp. Butter
1tsp Maple Syrup
¼ tsp. ginger or small chunk of fresh ginger
(to taste)
1 Cup Vegetable Broth
¼ Cup Cream (optional)
2 Onions, sautéed

Preheat oven to 350 degrees. Slice butternut squash lengthwise and remove seeds. Place the sides open face down on a cookie sheet. Use a fork to create steam holds on the skin of the squash, add some water to the pan and place into the oven. The squash is done when it can be easily pierced with a fork. Sauté onions in a little olive oil or butter. Scoop squash out of skin and add all ingredients to the blender until smooth.

~ *Garlicky Broth with Kale and Sweet Potatoes* ~

2 ½ tsp. Extra Virgin Olive Oil
1 Large Onion, chopped
3 ½ tsp. Italian Seasoning
6 Cups Vegetable Broth
2 15-oz Cans Cannellini Beans
1 lb. Sweet Potatoes (2-3 large), cut in chunks
10 Leaves Kale, removed from spine
12 Medium Garlic Cloves (9 if organic)

Heat oil in soup pot over medium heat. Add onion and seasonings and sauté until onion is soft and golden. Stir in broth, beans, sweet potatoes and bring to a boil. Reduce to low heat and simmer for 10 minutes. Add kale and garlic and simmer until potatoes are tender (10-15 minutes). Season with salt and pepper to taste.

~ *Egg Fried Rice* ~

2 Cups Brown Rice
4 Cups Water
1 Tbsp. Olive Oil (or Coconut Oil)
1 Cup Onions, chopped
2-3 Cloves Garlic, minced or sliced
1 Chunk Ginger Root, minced or sliced
3 Stalks Celery, chopped
1 Red or Yellow Pepper, chopped
½ Cup Carrots, grated
2 Eggs
2 Cups Greens (broccoli rabe, kale, spinach), chopped
Few tsps. Sesame Oil
Salt & Pepper
Optional: Tofu, Broccoli, Nuts or Seeds of choice

Cook brown rice in water until tender (about 40 min). Heat oil and sauté onions, garlic, ginger. Add celery, peppers and carrots and stir fry for 5-8 minutes. Add rice to vegetables and then crack the eggs on top and mix them in as they cook. Add greens last with a little sesame oil, salt and pepper to taste.

~ *Roasted Vegetables* ~

1 Rutabaga, peeled and chopped into
chunks
  5 Large Carrots, cut in thick slices
  2 Large Sweet Potatoes, cut into chunks
  1 Large Onion, peeled and cut into chunks
  Extra Virgin Olive Oil
  Salt and Pepper

Preheat oven to 450 degrees and place large
cookie sheet in the oven to warm. Place all
ingredients in large bowl and drizzle with
extra virgin olive oil, salt and pepper to taste.
Mix well and then pour vegetables onto heated
cookie sheet. After 15 minutes, mix the
vegetables around and cook for another 10-15
minutes until well done.

~ *Stuffed Dates* ~

10 Manjool Dates
20 Walnuts
Cinnamon
Salt

Cut dates in half, remove and discard the pits. Place a walnut or walnut pieces into each half. When complete, sprinkle dates with cinnamon and salt. Yum!

~ *Chia Pudding* ~

1 Cup Chia Seeds
½ Cup Coconut, grated
1 Tbsp Pure Maple Syrup
1 Cup Fresh Raspberries (or other berry)
3 Cups Milk of choice (Almond, Rice, Hemp)
Optional: Sunflower Seeds, Cacao or Carob Powder, Goji Berries, Chocolate Chips

Add all ingredients to a container you can vigorously shake. Shake, wait 10 minutes & repeat process 3x. Chia seeds may coagulate. Place in the fridge for a half hour or more. Enjoy!

~ *Apple Crisp* ~

10-12 Apples, sliced
4 Tbsp Pure Maple Syrup
2 Tbsp Cinnamon
½ Cup Raisins or Currants
1 Tbsp Almond Flour

Preheat oven to 375 degrees
Mix above ingredients together, layer into 9x12 baking dish.

Topping:
2 cups Gluten Free Oats
1 Cup Almond Flour
½ Cup Walnuts
1 Tbsp Cinnamon
½ Cup Pure Maple Syrup
½ Cup Melted Butter to make crumble

Mix topping ingredients together and place on top apple mixture.
Bake for 30 minutes covered and then 20 more minutes uncovered.

"You will never do anything in this world without courage. It is the greatest quality of the mind next to honor."

~ Aristotle ~

CHAPTER 20

So What's Next for You?

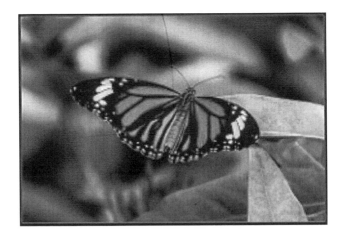

By now you know how many times I've started, stopped and started again. I'm guessing this is your story too. When you think about how often you get stuck in this cycle, do you feel helpless or worse, ashamed? Studies have shown how the rate of success increases when people have support and guidance when working through their challenges. If you've felt like this journey is overwhelming to do alone, I'm here for you.

Being able to confide in someone who understands what you are going through can make all the difference in life. Stress is the major factor impeding your health. Contributing to the stress may also be poor food choices and lack of exercise. Whatever your problem is, know that you do not need to handle it alone. Know that you are capable of changing your habits and that you are supported on your journey, I believe in you because I've been there!

This is not a one-size-fits-all life. We are each unique beings and that is why it is imperative that we each find our own way to optimal health. I've designed a program specifically for people just like you who want a course of action to help you recognize your strengths as well as areas that need improvement in your life. And you will finally be able to make lasting change that will positively impact your overall health and wellbeing. Life is full of stressors, so learning how to adapt to our environment or have the courage to change our environment is necessary to achieve lasting health.

Become educated around your food choices. I believe for most of us, making a change in our diets is the hardest thing to do. Remember you don't have to do it all at once, seek out the support you need to deal with these changes. There is a grieving process involved when you give up a staple food in your diet, even if it is only a temporary adjustment.

A good friend of mine once told me, "Bodies love to move!" And she is right, more than walking to the mailbox or out to the car, your body wants to be exercised. Sweating is healthy and it's time to find the right movement that will make your life more enjoyable.

And how do you make these changes last? We've all had temporary fixes before, but now it's time to make effective change. Health is indeed physical, it does have to do with what you eat and how much you exercise but it is also emotional as well as mental. These states of being effect your physical body, they effect your digestion and your immune system function. Gone are the days of believing our bodies are machines, we are holistic beings and we are deeply effected by our emotional states as well as our inner and outer environment.

If you are ready to make a significant change in your health and wellbeing, contact me for a complimentary *Healthier Living Breakthrough Session*. After this session you will be clear about your hidden stressors and the next steps to take to on your path to a more joyful living experience! Please contact me at trishbliss@me.com to schedule a session or book a speaking engagement.

Resources

Sugar Blues by William Dufty
Integrative Nutrition by Joshua Rosenthal
In Defense of Food by Michael Pollan
Body, Mind, Sport Dr. John Douillard
The Blood Sugar Solution by Dr. Mark Hyman

Overeaters Anonymous is a 12-Step based support group to help you recover from a sugar or food addiction. Check them out at OA.org